CONTENTS

INTRODUCTION

"I'm on a diet," you hear your friend say. A future of carrots and rabbit food pops into your mind. The truth is that weight is an issue a lot of us face. Obesity affected 93.3 million Americans in 2015 and 2016 according to the Center for Disease Control and Prevention. And in 2020, they reported that the number of people dieting has increased dramatically in the past 10 years alone. When we wanna drop a couple of pounds, or even 30 pounds, a harsh diet is usually the first thing we attempt. But diets don't always work, and can even set you back in your weight loss journey because of their restrictive nature. Let us tell you why, and what you can do instead to lose those extra pounds.

Our society for centuries now has applauded those with thin bodies and shamed those who are anything but. No matter what form of media we interact with, the concept of weight is construed to make us believe that our body isn't good enough. The media outlets that are targeted towards a young, particularly female, audience go out of their way to remind our girls that the only way they will be beautiful and accepted is if they fit into a size zero dress. A 2010 study revealed that girls as young as 3 years old are already preparing themselves to fit the thin ideal. Is this really what our society has come to? While in the past few years the Body Positivity social movement has made quite some improvements to the overall conversation around our bodies, we still have a long way to go.

WHY DIETS WON'T WORK

The Weight Loss Is Temporary

You give the newest trending diet a try and, after three months you've lost 30 pounds and you're feeling happy. Now that you've lost the weight you stop starving yourself, and go back to your normal eating habits. Suddenly you have gained *back* 35 pounds! This is an all too common problem. A 2007 study at UCLA done by Traci Mann, a UCLA associate professor of psychology found that "the majority of people [dieting] regained all the weight, plus more. Diets do not lead to sustained weight loss or health benefits for the majority of people." So even if you do suffer through a diet, it is very unlikely that the weight will remain off for long. Your weight loss becomes obsolete just like the thousands of diet plans out there. I know, it's unfair, but diets are only a short-term fix to a long-term problem.

Quote - "Up to 98% of people, according to research, regain all the weight that they lost within five years, and up to two-thirds of people end up regaining more weight than they lost," says anti-diet dietitian, Christy Harrison, M.P.H., R.D., C.D.N., author of *Anti-Diet* and host of the Food Psych podcast.

Diet Pundits And Their Dogmas

Every third person these days claims to be a diet pundit who knows everything there is to know about a "healthy" body and how to achieve it quickly. But frankly speaking, these so-called pundits are simply spreading misinformation regarding diets and healthy bodies they learned from other diet pundits. For example, a common dogma that these pundits parade around is that obesity is just an imbalance between the calories a person consumes and the calories they expend through their workouts. And let us tell you, this isn't necessarily true as there are a multitude of factors impacting our body, weight, and diet. So our advice to you is to not believe every diet pundit you encounter, instead speak to a dietician or nutritionist as they are better equipped to help you maintain a healthy body.

What Is Fat?

Fats are actually an essential macronutrient your body needs to function well and no matter the type of fat the amount of calories is the same – 9 Calories per gram. Yes, there are some bad fats, but there are also some good ones. Ever since people started spreading the word that "fat is bad," everyone has believed it without asking any questions. Many of your bodily functions depend on fat, and by depriving your body of all fat, you are putting yourself at risk. Essentially, fat is an energy source and a major source of calories. It protects your nerves and skeleton, allows other nutrients to function, provides warmth, builds cell membranes and hormones, increases absorption of fat-soluble vitamins (A,D,K & E), and increases energy. Depending on the type of fat, the effect it has on your health will differ accordingly especially when it comes to the health of your heart and blood. But keep in mind, there are certain fats that are not as beneficial for your body. Knowing the difference is key.

- Saturated Fats
  - Raises cholesterol levels, specifically low-density lipoprotein, or "bad," cholesterol

- Increases the risk of cardiovascular diseases and stroke
    - Found in dairy products, meats, baked goods, etc.
    - Maximum 13 grams per day is recommended by the American Heart Association
  - Unsaturated Fats
    - Supports good health
    - Maintains levels of high-density lipoprotein, or "good," cholesterol
    - Different forms – Monounsaturated or Polyunsaturated
    - Found in oils, nuts, seeds, etc.
  - Trans Fats or Partially Hydrogenated Oils
    - Manufactured
    - Not at all essential to the body because of its damaging effects
    - Increases levels of low-density cholesterol
    - Decreases levels of high-density cholesterol
    - High risk for heart diseases, type 2 diabetes, and stroke
    - Provide certain food products with a longer shelf life
    - Found in fried foods, pastries, pies, pizza dough, shortenings, packaged foods, etc.

Fats also come in different forms based on their attributes.

- Fats or Fatty Acids – solids at room temperature
- Oils – liquids at room temperature
- Lipids – solid or liquid at room temperature
- Vegetable Fats – fats usually found in vegetables like avocados, olives, peanuts, etc.
- Animal Fats – fats that come from animals such as cream, butter, lard, etc.

Food Becomes The Enemy

Taking the pleasure out of anything can make life difficult. Now if you take it a step further, and begin to demonize an object, it can start to influence the way you think. Diets often tell us fat is evil, don't even look at carbs, and sugar is the enemy. These diet mantras have real consequences and can trigger many eating disorders. According to the National Eating Disorder Association using a diet to lose weight can lead to anorexia, orthorexia, bulimia, binge eating, and more. Diet culture in general perpetuates the idea that gaining weight is bad. PERIOD. Our Instagram feeds are filled with posts by already skinny or fit people telling us how they dropped 20 pounds in a week by doing juice cleanses or fasting or cutting out some food item or the other. None of which are healthy methods to practice because of the toll it takes on your body.

Atkins, Paleo, Whole30, South Beach, basically any fad diet promises a snatched waistline, but it is at the cost of necessary nutrients. Western culture has in the past decade or so normalized diet culture without even realizing that in certain ways they are glorifying disordered eating behaviors. According to the National Eating Disorder Association, 35% of dieting turns obsessive. And of that 35%, 20 to 25% turns into an eating disorder.

The Problem With Low-Fat Diets

When it comes to weight loss, people are so quick to turn to quick fixes that they don't often realize the consequences it can have on their body. Low-fat diets for instance restrict people so that only 30% of their daily Calorie intake is composed of fat. However, there have been studies that claimed that low-fat diets are not the most efficient when it comes to long term weight loss.

Ultra-low-fat diets are even more detrimental as they allow only 10% of your Calories to come from fat. It is also quite high in carbohydrates and low in protein. These types of diets are mainly plant-based so your intake of animal products like meat, eggs, dairy, etc. is limited to a certain extent. Food items such as nuts, extra virgin olive oil, and avocados, which are considered high-fat plant food, are also restricted. As we mentioned, fat is essential for your body because of its many functions. With these diets, you lose your necessary fat which harms your body. The main thing to keep in mind is that any food item in excess is unhealthy. So yes, you can practice a low-fat diet, but not to the extreme where your health suffers.

While low-fat diets have their downside, they can actually be good for your overall health if administered properly.

- Heart Disease
    - Low-fat diets can control blood pressure, blood cholesterol, and C-reactive protein
- Type 2 Diabetes
    - Low-fat diets can decrease a patient's need for insulin therapy
- Obesity
    - Aids weight loss
- Multiple Sclerosis
    - Can slow the progression of the disease and its effects

Your Metabolism Slows Down

It's true that you must be in a caloric deficit to lose weight. This means that your body must burn more calories than it consumes. Dieting often forces your body to slow down or conserve energy. Especially when you stop eating, or eat too little, your metabolism will take a hit. According to research, when you're on a severely low-calorie diet your body overcompensates by slowing down your metabolism. Meaning that over time you will start to burn fewer calories. "Yo-yo" dieting (losing weight and gaining weight in a repetitive cycle), especially, impacts your metabolism negatively. You must keep a moderate diet or else you will lose weight at a slower rate or stop losing weight altogether.

Diets Mess With Hunger Cues

When you diet, a lot of your time is spent ignoring your body's hunger cues. This makes you less responsive to hunger cues in the future, and eventually makes it harder to regulate your weight. Our bodies then become confused about when we should or should not be eating. You can begin to overeat, eat because of boredom, or have emotional eating issues. Instead of teaching people to recognize the difference between emotional hunger and physical hunger, the dieting mindset urges people to ignore their body's hunger cues no matter what. So essentially, if your stomach is growling you should see it as a good thing because by not feeding yourself you are somehow doing yourself a favor. All these diet pundits say that most of the time you are not really hungry but just bored which is completely incorrect and a dangerous thing to constantly repeat. Especially when it comes to women, these so-called experts claim that women should not eat too much like men and should instead watch their diet. Really?! You should be able to trust your body and the signs it gives you without questioning it or feeling guilty. When you get on any new diet plan, you get one step closer to ruining your relationship with your body. These diet plans are innately designed to teach you to somehow "outsmart" your hunger which is unhealthy for your mind and your body. Remember your hunger is not your enemy.

Overeating

When you are stressing about your diet and not allowing yourself to eat foods you enjoy, you increase your stress hormone known as cortisol. Cortisol has been linked to overeating and can cause your insulin levels to rise and blood sugar to drop. This makes you crave sweets and junk food that you can't have on a diet. Thus, begins a cruel cycle of calorie restriction and craving that creates a perfect recipe for a downfall. We all have our weakness when it comes to food and there is nothing wrong with that. However, when we lose our control it becomes an issue that can be quite risky. Media platforms that preach diet plans and weight loss and summer body goals often associate our favorite foods with weight gain. We, too, begin to feel guilty the moment we come in contact with these foods because there's a voice constantly reminding us that even a bit of that chocolate cake will make you fat.

You Are Never Satisfied

No matter how much you diet and lose weight, you somehow are never satisfied with your weight. Once you reach that certain number on the scale, you instantly aim for a lower one. It is an ever-present goal. Diet culture preaches that following any diet will leave you feeling amazing simply because you have a 36-24-24 figure. But in reality that is not true because in order to achieve that figure you essentially put your body through hell. Speaking from experience, being on a diet is exhausting. Your body is deprived of essential nutrients and constantly working to keep you functioning. After a while, even completing simple daily tasks becomes too much to handle. And let's get one thing straight, there is no such thing as the "right" body size. We live in a society that advocates for body positivity while simultaneously pressurizing people to invest in the diet industry which is already worth at least $71 billion. So you spend money on all these diets, "skinny" teas, waist trainers, etc. but you cost yourself your self-respect and worth.

Skinny Does Not Equate Healthy

There is an assumption by the general population that people who are skinny are healthier than those who are not. However, that is not necessarily true. A research team led by Ruth Loos in 2011 found that lean people who have a specific genetic variant – IRS1 – were actually more likely to develop type 2 diabetes and heart diseases. They examined the genetic code of at least 75,000 people before coming to this conclusion. Fat is stored differently amongst people and it is mostly dependent on genes and gender. For example, with lean individuals there is no visible body fat; however, it could be stored around their organs and in the muscles. Just because you look skinny it does not mean that you are immune to health issues. It is highly recommended that you practice a nutritious, active lifestyle regardless of what your body size is.

The Problem With Spot Reduction Workouts

We have all clicked on those two-week ab challenge videos or one week arm challenge ones or muffin top challenges. Especially with summer just around the corner, these types of workout videos are littered through social media. The main idea of these spot reduction exercises is that they claim to reduce body fat in specific areas of your body. For instance, doing a hundred sit ups will give you a flatter stomach or doing fifty prayer pulses will reduce your flabby arms. But in reality, there is no real evidence that proves that spot reduction actually works.

See, when you want to lose weight, you have to go into a calorie deficit which means that you must expend more calories than you consume. During this process, your body uses energy which is stored in your cells in the form of fat. Your body shape becomes smaller as there is less stored fat. However, it is important to know that your body does not draw the required energy only from the specific areas you target during these workouts. So if you are working your abdominal area, your body is not just drawing the stored fat from there. It draws energy from the whole body. Yes, specific exercises can make those areas stronger and more toned, but they won't necessarily remove all the fat stored there. Instead of putting all your time and energy into these workouts, choose compound exercise which works multiple body parts at once. Planks, push-ups, squats, deadlifts, pull ups, etc. are all great examples of compound exercises that effectively work more muscles and, in turn, burn more fat.

Even if you want to lose weight in a certain area of your body, you have to approach it holistically. You have to work your whole body so that you can tone down proportionally. And that's not all, you have to also be mindful of your nutritional intake. You can't expect a toned body when your diet mostly consists of fried or frozen meals. Weight loss of any kind is a comprehensive process with many layers. In order for you to successfully change your body to your liking, nutrition and exercise are equally important.

WHAT DOES WORK?

Make Your Own Meals

The best way to maintain a healthy lifestyle is to cook your own food. When you do this, you can see exactly what is going into your meals, and you can control your own portions. Restaurants give massive serving sizes, and often fill the food with sugar and other ingredients that are unhealthy in these quantities. Preparing your own meals means that you are in control. You can gage how much you are eating, and you get a better handle on your food habits.

Given how busy everyone's schedule is these days, you can even try out meal prepping and see how that works for you. It is a great tool that makes meal time so much easier and it keeps you on track for healthy eating. Sometimes when we are short on time or exhausted from a long day at work, we most often end up eating out which are often high in calories and other forms of harmful fats. Here is a basic outline of meal planning looks like:

- Decide your meals – Before you even go to the grocery store, make a list of the meals you will make that week and decide what ingredients you need. If it helps, make a spreadsheet and write it all down. The key thing is to stay organized.
- Go shopping – Make a grocery list and go to the store, but make sure not to let your eyes and hands wander. Stick to the list.

- Prep work – Cook things like proteins and whole grains first as they take longer. And if you don't like to cook your food items ahead of time, just marinate them so they are ready to go on the day. You can also cook these items in large batches so you have enough for multiple meals.
- Chop fresh produce – To avoid spending too much time chopping vegetables and fruits, keep them cut beforehand and store them properly.
- Repeat meals – Assign each day a specific meal. For example, taco Tuesday or Mediterranean Wednesday.

We know it can be hard to choose home cooked meals over takeout especially when they are just a few clicks away. Cooking is a very intimate activity and it opens up many avenues for you to relax and reconnect with your loved ones. Whether it be through sharing old recipes or creating new ones, cooking at home is bound to make your heart and your stomach happy. Cooking at home also makes it easier for you to maintain a healthy, balanced diet. Takeout foods are often filled with unnecessary ingredients that make you consume more calories than you need without providing your body the right nutrients. At restaurants, the meals are often high in sodium, saturated fats, total fats, etc. All of which are detrimental to your health in excess. And trust, takeout meals multiple times a week add up real quick. Making sure that your meals have fresh ingredients will do wonders for your body and it will show. Since you are in charge of what does and doesn't go in your food, it is much easier to watch your calories, especially if you are trying to maintain a calorie deficit. And it's not like you have to count the calories of every ingredient or even figure out its nutritional value. Many recipes these days, whether online or in print, come with all the nutritional information you need including the calories and serving size. Especially if your schedule is hectic with work, hobbies, family, travel, etc., making your meals at home can actually save you a lot of time if you meal prep ahead of time. When you think about it, take-out actually takes about an hour to finally get to your table. And if you are ordering during rush hour, it is even later. So to avoid any hangry showdowns, it is better to be your own chef, waiter, and delivery man.

If you are one of those people who isn't as confident in their culinary skills and survives mostly on toast, we've got you covered. We recommend using food services like Hello Fresh, Daily Harvest, Blue Apron, Sakara Life, etc. These are some great organizations with weekly, monthly, and even annual subscriptions that deliver fresh ingredients, meal kits, and recipes straight to your home. All you have to do is follow the instructions and your food will be ready in no time.

Mindful Eating

Sometimes we order a large pizza, and we intend to eat it over the course of a weekend. But then we turn on *Jane The Virgin* and suddenly the whole pizza is gone. Mindful eating is a technique which helps people eat just enough to provide their body with the required fuel. It means being present when you sit down to enjoy a meal. When you eat, eat with your undivided attention. That way you don't overeat. Not that you can't turn on the T.V. when you are enjoying a snack on a Friday night, but it shouldn't be a habit. Mindful eating also entails enjoying your food thoroughly. Take each bite one at a time and chew slowly. If it helps, place your utensils down after every bite. The main purpose of this practice is to aid in weight loss, decrease binge eating of any kind, recognize hunger cues, engage your senses, and to help you foster a better relationship with food. If you think about it, it is almost like a type of meditation. In today's day and age, televisions and smartphones are constantly around us, especially during mealtimes. And its starts from a very young age when parents allow their kids to watch television just so they can finish their food quickly. Constantly growing in this environment, we get habituated to the process of eating while watching something. Eating so mindlessly is highly problematic especially given the fact that your brain needs about 20 minutes to signal that the stomach is full. That's what often happens with binge eating because by the time you realize you are full, you already ate too much. Mindful eating is an important practice to incorporate in your life because it helps you distinguish between emotional and physical hunger cures.

Here are some tips to keep in mind when you start practicing mindful eating:

- Chew thoroughly
- Put down your utensils after a few bites
- Eliminate any distractions
- Eat in silence
- Understand how the food makes you feel

We know that changes can be difficult and even uncomfortable sometimes, so to start maybe try this for just one meal a day.

Follow The Hunger Pendulum

If you think about it, your body's appetite system works almost like a pendulum which swings between hunger and fullness. On each side there is an extreme – one being the various levels of fullness and the other being the rising levels of hunger. When you are eating, the pendulum swings closer and closer towards fullness. Over the course of the next few hours, it swings in the other direction towards hunger.

In instances when you overeat, you consume more than what your body needs to produce the energy to keep your body functioning; thus, the pendulum is at the fullness extreme. Your body also ends up taking longer to use up that excess food into energy. You may have said to yourself after a large lunch that you will skip dinner or eat light. But by the time dinner comes around, your hunger is triggered again just by the thought of delicious food or even the timing. Your hunger pendulum then gets pushed further and further towards fullness. You may have noticed that in these instances, the food does not always taste as good. This is because when you are already full and continue to eat, your taste buds don't react as much. They are only sensitive to taste when your body needs the food.

On the other hand, when you reach the point of starvation your body becomes too weak to even signal that you are hungry. You also end up overeating in these situations because your body has been deprived of food for too long. The pendulum, as a consequence, sprints in the opposite direction. That is why dietary restrictions of any kind are harmful. It entails tremendous psychological and physiological pressure when it comes to meals. Most diets fail because of this and even lead to eating disorders. Your appetite pendulum is unique to your body, so listen to it.

Stop Counting Your Calories

One of the side effects of diet culture is the obsessive nature people have towards calories in their food. There's more to it than simply burning more calories than you consume. Dr. Fatima Cody Stanford is an obesity specialist and assistant professor of medicine and pediatrics at the Harvard Medical School who says, "'This idea of 'a calorie in and a calorie out' when it comes to weight loss is not only antiquated, it's just wrong.'" There are many factors at play when it comes to how your body actually burns calories – your body's metabolism, what foods you consume, gut microbiome, etc. When people say that every body is different, they are not lying. Two people can consume the same number of calories yet have different outcomes in terms of their weight.

- Metabolism – Your body is governed by a "set point" which is different for everyone. And this set point is a combination of many factors such as your genes, your behaviors, your environment, etc. To make sure that your body doesn't drop below this set point, your hypothalamus keeps you in check. So no matter how much you diet and exercise, your body will not allow you to go past the minimum.

- Food Types – We cannot stress this enough but not all food is created equal. Whatever food choices you make influence your calorie intake. *Cell Metabolism* published a study in 2019 which concluded that people who eat processed foods are more likely to eat more calories compared to those who eat unprocessed foods. While it's okay to eat processed foods sometimes, you should keep in mind that it spikes your calorie intake so you should avoid it as much as possible.
- Gut Microbiome – Your gut hosts trillions of organisms and some of the major ones influence how many calories you actually absorb. Studies have shown that certain organisms reside in those who are naturally thin. And these organisms differ from those who are naturally overweight. Dr. Stanford says, "'Taking the gut microbiota out of people who are lean and placing it in people who have overweight or obesity can result in weight shifts.'"

Give Yourself A Break

Do you want something sweet? Have some berries. If you really want the chocolate cake - have it. Don't deny yourself pleasure, we all want happiness and joy. Having a few meals here and there won't make you a terrible person. And don't even consider these "cheat" meals because that terminology itself is problematic. It carries such a negative connotation and makes people feel like they need to punish themselves at the gym the next day for it. Same goes for your day-to-day meals. Try to avoid labelling foods as "good" or "bad." Yes, some food items are not beneficial for your body but that doesn't make it your enemy. If you are constantly invested in these labels, you can easily turn a minor slip-up into a catastrophe. It is completely okay to make mistakes and get back on track the next day. One meal won't make it or break it for you. A piece of cake a week won't kill you, and it won't throw off your weight loss. But a piece of cake *every* night, plus a muffin in the morning is a different story. Just be mindful of the food choices you are making. And at the end of the day, it is about balance.

Indulging in these "happy" meals can actually be beneficial for your body because they help restore the hormone leptin in your body. This hormone works to keep your energy levels balanced and it signals your brain to stop eating when the stomach is full. It also helps boost your metabolism. Many psychologists and nutritionists have found that such "happy" meals satisfy your cravings and even encourage you to stick to your diet plan. For example, if you are trying to achieve a calorie deficit it can be difficult to stop yourself from eating that chocolate bar or that slice of cheesecake. But if you allow yourself to indulge once in a while, your body will start to habituate to it. And then you won't be so prone to having those empty calories just for the fun of it only to regret it later.

The Idea Of Calorie Deficit

Let us start from the basics, the units of energy you receive from the food you consume is known as calories. When you burn less calories compared to how much you are consuming, your body goes through calorie deficit. The amount of calories you burn daily are split into three components: resting energy expenditure, thermic effect of food, and activity energy expenditure.

- Resting energy expenditure – These are the calories your body burns while your body is at rest and performing basic functions such as breathing or blood circulation.
- Thermic effect of food – These are the calories your body burns while digesting and metabolizing the food you eat.
- Activity energy expenditure – These are the calories you burn while exercising and basically doing anything that involves movement.

It is recommended that we should ideally eat about 2,000 calories worth of food daily. In a calorie deficit, it is enough to just reduce your calorie intake by 500 calories per day to see change in your body composition. This number is good because it helps you maintain your fitness goals without putting your body at a risk of any kind. When you are just starting to practice calorie deficit, you should know what your maintenance calories are beforehand. Maintenance calories are the calories your body needs to keep your body functioning properly so that it can allow you to be active throughout the day. There are different ways to do this: use the Body Weight Planner by the National Institute of health or calculate your calories for 10 days.

- Calculating maintenance calories – Track your calories using a tracking app and weigh yourself everyday while maintaining your daily activity levels. If you want more accurate results, wear the same clothes and measure yourself at the same time on the same scale. It is normal for your weight to fluctuate from day to day. But overall, your weight should have remained about the same over the course of the 10 days and the average amount of calories you consumed each day will give a better representation of your maintenance calories. To calculate this average daily calorie intake number, divide your total calories consumed over the ten days by ten. Then, subtract 500 and now you have your new daily calorie intake goal. Remember though, as you begin to notice your weight loss, your maintenance calories will also begin to go down over time. So keep adjusting your calories intake. It is dangerous to consume less than 1,200 calories per day.

There are multiple ways you can achieve a calorie deficit. You can either consume fewer calories as we mentioned or increase your physical activity throughout the day. You can even try out both if you have the time and energy for it. But for most people, it might be easier to maintain a calorie deficit through their diet alone. With exercise it is a bit difficult to keep up because somedays you just don't have the motivation, you might not feel well, you might not have enough time in your schedule, you might be travelling, etc. And anyways, it is much easier to eat 500 calories less everyday than burn them. You don't need to worry about making drastic changes to your diet and grocery list when it comes to maintaining a calorie deficit. Even the smallest things will make a large impact. Here are some tips to keep in mind:

- Avoid drinking your calories – It will be a lot easier for you to reach that target of eating 500 fewer calories if you start by just eliminating any sugary drinks in your diet such as soda, juices, special coffee drinks, alcohol, etc. That's not to say that you can never have them but try to limit them as much as possible because they don't offer much to your overall health.
- Limit your consumption of highly processed foods – highly processed foods like sugary beverages, desserts, and fast foods are irresistible but also high in calories because of their fat, sugar, and salt content. It's like once you start you can't stop.
- Eat minimally processed foods – try to fill your diet with mostly minimally processed foods which are rich in minerals, vitamins, and fiber. These foods prevent you from overeating while making sure that your body gets its required nutrients.
- Eat mostly home-cooked meals – one of the easiest ways to control your calorie intake is to make your meals at home. Not only can you practice a calorie deficit, but you can also choose more nutritious ingredients and your portion size. A study conducted in 2015 found that those who had home cooked meals at least six to seven times per week actually consumed 137 fewer calories daily compared to those who only ate at home once or twice.

Intuitive Eating

The concept of intuitive eating has been around since the mid-90s when it was first introduced by dietitians Elyse Resch and Evelyn Tribole. It is essentially an "anti-diet" as it helps you establish a method of mindfully eating without guilt or food restrictions and understanding your body's hunger signals. Think of it as rehab for chronic dieters. The main purpose of the intuitive eating style is to encourage a healthy relationship with food and body image. This style of eating teaches you to only eat when you are hungry and to stop when you are full. And while this may seem like an intuitive process, many people struggle with this because they are so consumed by diet culture. This disrupts the relationship people share with their body as they trust the diet pundits more than their body's signals. You have to understand that *how* you eat is equally as important as *what* you eat.

A main part of this eating style is to relearn trusting your body, which begins with differentiating between emotional and physical hunger.

- Emotional Hunger – This hunger is usually driven by your emotional needs. Emotions like stress, anxiety, sadness, loneliness, etc. can cause cravings for comfort foods like ice cream, chocolate, cookies, etc. And after giving in to your cravings, you often feel guilty and start bringing yourself down for eating such foods.
- Physical Hunger – This hunger is really your biological urge to recharge with necessary nutrients. There are many signals of this hunger such as fatigue, irritability, or a growling stomach. The only way to satisfy it is by consuming food.

The philosophy of intuitive eating has 10 key principles

- Reject the Diet Mentality
- Honor Your hunger
- Make Peace with Food
- Challenge the Food Police
- Discover the Satisfaction Factor
- Feel Your Fullness
- Cope with Your Emotions with Kindness
- Respect Your Body
- Movement – Feel the Difference
- Honor Your Health – Gentle Nutrition

While research on the benefits of intuitive eating is still ongoing, studies so far show that it leads to a lower body mass index, weight maintenance (not to be mixed with weight loss), and healthier mindset in general. When we confine ourselves within a specific diet plan, our mental health often takes a hit. However, intuitive eating reverses those effects. In fact, many participants who have been a part of intuitive eating studies claimed that the eating style built their self-esteem, improved their body image issues, decreased depression or anxiety, and encouraged a healthier attitude towards life. In terms of eating disorders, the more you actively practice intuitive eating the less likely you are to suffer from any such disorders.

So if you're ready to break up with diet culture, get started on your intuitive eating journey.

Protein Loading

Like carbohydrates and fat, protein is another such macronutrient that is essential for your body because of its many functions. In order to benefit from the nutrients protein has, you have to keep track of when you are consuming it so that it works in your body's favor. The best times to protein-load are right after workouts, afternoon to evening, and during the offseason.

- After Workouts - Consuming protein after your workouts is beneficial because it works to repair any damage your muscles suffered through during the workout at a faster pace. The main purpose is to simply ensure that your muscles repair properly.
- Afternoon to Evening - The reason why it is recommended to have protein late in the day is because that is when your body needs it most. During the day your body requires carbohydrates as it is the most active part of the day. As the day progresses, your body switches to repair/regeneration mode and that is where protein comes in.
- Offseason - This is mostly for athletes who participate in race-focused training such as endurance athletes. Such athletes should increase their protein intake in the few weeks before they start their next training cycle. This helps reduce muscle loss and increase fat loss. Once you

start your training, you should switch back to focusing on carbohydrates for the energy.

Increasing your protein intake can slow down your appetite, increase fat burning, and help you gain muscle. Can it get better than that?! Your protein of choice doesn't have to be chicken or red meat either. Lentils, chickpeas, and quinoa are all healthy vegetarian-friendly protein options that even carnivores will love. But as always, anything in excess will only harm your body and you only need a little bit of protein to experience its benefits.

Stay Active For You

With so much stress on having the perfect body, many people begin to lose interest in exercising and staying active. Working out becomes a punishment and we begin to despise even the thought of it. And let's be honest, we all have had those times where we have promised to complete that two-week shred challenge but ended up giving up on the fourth third day. It's okay you can admit it. There is no shame because we are all in the same boat. But there is no need to be discouraged because it is not really our fault. No matter what workout trend we jump on and attempt to complete, we almost always give up when we realize that we cannot perform the moves "perfectly." All the workout videos for such weeklong trends are often conducted by fit, lean people who can easily do the moves. When we attempt to do the same, we get discouraged seeing them do sit ups without breaking a sweat while we struggle to even lift our back off the mat. We can't seem to accept the idea that when we workout it is for fun and there is no need to be perfect at it. Why does working out have to feel like a momentous task?

Everyone's fitness journey is unique to their body. That yoga instructor on your television who is doing the crow pose so effortlessly has years of experience supporting them. They did not just wake up one morning magically knowing how to do the pose perfectly. The purpose of exercise or any form of active movement for that matter is to simply keep our heart, mind, and body healthy. So why do we complicate such a simple thing? Honestly speaking, the phrase "practice makes perfect" does not do much to help people because they are more focused on perfection. Instead, we recommend saying "practice makes progress." It is an undemanding philosophy that encourages you to practice for yourself. It opens up a whole new space where you can confidently make mistakes and learn from them. Especially with exercise, you need to allow your body to figure things out on its own and learn to understand what it wants.

Here are some fun physical activity ideas you can try:

- Frisbee
- Jump rope
- Dance class
- Hiking
- Rock Climbing
- Hula hoop
- Orienteering
- Cycling
- Slacklining
- Pole dancing
- Gardening
- Walk dogs

Cardio Vs. Strength Training

When it comes to weight loss, many people are quick to jump on the treadmill and run their feet off while others hit the weights. Both parties are right in their own way because they are working their bodies in specific ways and ultimately shedding some weight or toning up. But let's break down the difference between cardio training and strength/weight training so that you have a better understanding of what works best for you.

Cardio exercise of any kind helps your body burn more calories per session. Research has revealed that people can estimate the number of calories they are likely to burn during their workouts based on their body weight. So for example, a person that weighs 160 pounds, would burn about 250 calories for every 30 minutes of moderate paced jogging. And if they were to increase the pace to let's say six miles per hour, they would burn about 365 calories in the same time. But if they were doing weight training for 30 minutes, they might only burn between 130-220 calories. Basically, the number of calories you burn exercising depends on not only your body size but also on the intensity of your workouts.

While cardio burns more calories per session, strength training makes you burn more calories per day amongst other benefits. Cardio is good for your body, but it does not help you build and tone your muscles which burns calories even at rest. Thus, many people recommend strength training for weight loss because it is essential to increasing your resting metabolism by a few percent. Not only that, but your calorie also burning capacity isn't just limited to your strength training session. Research shows that you actually continue burning calories in the hours after your session.

High-Intensity Interval Training or HIIT is another style of workout that has similar benefits to a cardio session but in comparatively less time. A HIIT session can last between ten to thirty minutes and it consists of various intervals of short, intense workouts followed by low-intensity recovery workouts. We've had some experience with HIIT workouts and we highly recommend it. There are many great YouTube videos out there that you can watch and follow along. And it is totally okay to not be able to do the workouts perfectly, we sure struggled the first few days. Some instructors even offer modifications that still work your body while also looking out for it. Because these exercises are conducted in short intervals, it makes the time go by even faster.

These are just a few of the options you can try out to begin your fitness journey. The key thing to remember is that make sure you surprise your body with different exercises every day. If you do the same thing every day, your body gets used to it and your body adjusts to it. Then you are more likely to hit a weight loss plateau, so switch it up here and there. Your main goal is to keep your body moving every day. You don't have to work out till your body is sore and soaked in sweat. Give yourself and your muscles a few days to recharge and relax.

Take Up Yoga

Spending hours at the gym lifting weights or running on the treadmill is not something everyone enjoys or even has the time for with their busy schedules. And there is no shame in not going to the gym because at the end of the day it is a personal choice. As long as you are keeping your body active and healthy, it doesn't really matter whether the work is taking place at a gym or in your basement.

Yoga is one of those few exercises that anyone and everyone can do, that too anywhere. It is an instant natural way to heal your body with almost no equipment other than your body and determination. The mental and physical health benefits of yoga are unmatched.

- Improves balance, strength, and flexibility – Deep breathing and slow, steady movements warm up your muscles while also increasing your blood flow. Your body builds strength as it learns to support you while you hold poses for longer periods of time.
  - Try: Tree Pose, Downward Dog, Half Moon Pose
- Eases back pain – When it comes to any sort of body pain such as chronic back pain, the first-line treatment that is recommended by many physicians is almost always yoga. It stretches your muscles, relaxes your body, and improves mobility all at once.
  - Try: Cat-Cow Pose, Extended Triangle, Sphinx

Pose
- Good for heart health – Practicing yoga on a regular basis is quite beneficial for you because it reduces stress levels in the body as well as inflammation, which promotes a healthy heart. There are many yoga asanas, or poses, that decrease blood pressure and control body weight.
  - Try: Downward Dog, Bridge Pose, Bow Pose
- Promotes better sleep – Many studies have found that practicing yoga for a few minutes before going to sleep can improve the quality of your sleep.
  - Try: Legs Up the Wall Pose, Wide Knee Child's Pose, Corpse Pose
- Control stress levels – Yoga is known for not only its physical benefits but also for its mental health and spiritual benefits too. Even a few minutes every day can help bring some calmness into your life.
  - Try: Corpse Pose, Child's Pose, Standing Forward Fold Pose
- Weight management, increased metabolism, and toning – Although yoga is not a traditional aerobic exercise per say, there are more intense forms of yoga, like power yoga or vinyasa, that increase the amount of calories you burn to help you shed some weight. You should perform these practices at least three to five times per week.
  - Try: Sun Salutations, Boat Pose, Plank Pose

Stretch... Everyday

To protect your body's mobility and overall functionality, it is crucial that you stretch your muscles on a daily basis. As we get older, a lot of us experience joint pain, weakness in our limbs, lack of flexibility, and various other physical ailments. In order to maintain good health, stretching for even five minutes a day is enough. If we don't, our muscles become stiff and shorten which can lead to strains, muscle damage, and joint pains. Especially in this time of zoom meetings, sitting in a chair all day long tightens our hamstrings, knees, legs, and even causes back pain. You cannot just go from sitting down for eight hours straight to sprinting or cycling. The sudden pressure caused by such strenuous activities injures your muscles as they are not strong enough. Yes, it may seem overwhelming at first given that we have so many muscles, but it is not necessary to stretch each and every single one. Just work on the more important ones that you use on a daily basis. These critical areas are mostly composed of the lower half of your body such as your calves, your hamstrings, your hip flexors, etc. Remember stretching once in a whole won't do you any good. Your muscles have become tight because of months and even years of limited movement, so it won't go away in a matter of minutes. Consistency is key and that is what is going to help your body.

Here are some stretches you can daily to get you started:

- Downward dog
- Side oblique stretch
- Crescent pose
- Child's pose
- Figure 4
- Cat -Cow
- Forward fold
- Back twists
- Triceps stretch
- Frog stretch

Quote – "A lot of people don't understand that stretching has to happen on a regular basis. It should be daily," says David Nolan, a physical therapist at Harvard-affiliated Massachusetts General Hospital.

Take Care Of Your Gut

Although there are no "skinny" bacteria out there that will magically flatten your stomach, the bacteria that resides in your gut plays a critical role in regulating your metabolism, absorbing nutrients well, and managing your body weight. The large intestine is home to trillions of microbes which compose your gut microbiota. And the more diverse your microbiome is, the more beneficial it is for your overall health. The goal is to make sure that your intestinal environment is balanced so that it does not lead to dysbiosis, which means that your body lacks beneficial bacteria. Individuals who are obese or overweight usually show patterns of dysbiosis. And this is often connected to inflammation and a higher blood sugar level because more energy is being extracted from the food you consume. The Western diet, for instance, leads to obesity and dysbiosis because it is so high in sugar and fat. Just like your weight, a balanced, healthy lifestyle will keep your gut health in check.

Akkermansia muciniphila and Christensenella are two bacteria that are considered "good" gut bacteria. They are also associated with lean bodies as they help prevent unnecessary weight gain.

- Akkermansia – strengthens your intestinal barrier by feeding on the mucus that lines the gut. It also produces a short-chain fatty acid known as acetate which regulates body fat storage as well as appetite.
- Christensenella – helps with weight control and is also present in lean individuals. The interesting thing about this microbe is that it is related to your genetic makeup. So if your relatives had it, you are more likely to have it too. There are some people who don't have any and that is normal too.

The American Gut Project found that people with the greatest microbiota diversity ate plant foods of various colors throughout the week. So make sure to fill your plate with as many colors as you can at each meal. This is why many people recommend a natural plant-based diet these days. It has numerous health benefits such as reducing your calories intake, aiding weight loss, lowering metabolic markers, and nourishing gut bacteria as many plants have various prebiotic fibers.

- Red – Anti-inflammatory, supports immune system, full of antioxidants
    - cherry, red onion, tomato, apple, cranberry
- Yellow – Full of antioxidants, promotes healthy gut microbiome, decreases blood sugar, increases gastric

emptying
  ◦ Banana, ginger, lemon, corn
- Orange – Fertility, many healthy gut bacteria, full of anti-oxidants
  ◦ Orange, mango, carrot, apricot, turmeric
- Green – Promotes healthy blood circulation, antioxidant properties, many healthy gut bacteria
  ◦ Olive, green apple, cabbage, artichoke

Believe it or not, your gut health is also impacted by how much time you invest in physical activity. Those who lead a sedentary lifestyle are more likely to have a less diverse microbiome compared to those who are more active. You can increase the amount of health-promoting bacteria, such as Akkermansia muciniphila, in your gut with simple aerobic exercises like walking, swimming, dancing, cycling etc. The more you move your body the more stable your metabolic markers will be.

Visual Tricks

This next one is a clever trick that works on your brain's perception. Grab a smaller plate than normal but keep your portion size the same. This makes the plate look fuller, and our brain believes that it is eating more food than normal. Too often, especially in American culture, we eat past our point of being full. Using a smaller plate helps train our bodies to recognize when we are satisfied.

Stay Hydrated

Nothing, I REPEAT, nothing is more important than staying hydrated. Our brains often mistake thirst for hunger, leading us to reach for a bag of chips when we should be filling our cups at the sink. Drinking water keeps your skin clear, your energy up, boosts your metabolism, and makes you feel full. When you are dehydrated, your energy levels are quite low and you can easily skip your workouts. To eliminate fats more efficiently from your system, you should drink at least 8 cups of water daily.

Some quick tips to make sure that you are hydrated:

- Carry a water bottle everywhere
- Implement water into your daily routine
- Hydrate before you exercise
- Add some lemon slices or fruits to add some flavor to your water
- Drink herbal teas

Sleep

Sleep is the second most crucial item on this list. Not sleeping enough, at least 8 hours, can mess with the levels of our hormones ghrelin and leptin. This hormone imbalance makes us more likely to gain weight, even if we are leading a healthy life. High-quality sleep is key and it is dependent on many factors such as the amount of exercise we get, time we spend on our electronics, exposure to sun, and the types of food and drinks we consume among other things. Ana Krieger, MD, MPH, Medical Director of the Center for Sleep Medicine at New York Presbyterian and Weill Cornell Medicine claims that our brain health and activity, our sleep for instance, are highly impacted by a nutrient-rich diet. A recent study found that your sleep is more likely to suffer when you eat less fiber, more sugar, and more saturated fats. "Eating healthy and allowing the body to absorb proper nutrients provides the brain with the chemical environment that it needs to produce the neurotransmitters that it needs to maintain adequate sleep," Krieger says. The nutrients we get from food serve as the building blocks for other minerals and proteins that are needed to create the amino acids that are involved in sleep, she says.

 If you are not sleeping well or at odd times, it can negatively impact your circadian rhythm which is your body's 24-hour cycle. The circadian rhythm makes sure that your body is functioning on time. Kristin Eckel-Mahan, PhD, Assistant Professor at the

Center for Metabolic and Degenerative Diseases at The University of Texas Health Science Center of Houston says that we can actually reprogram the many clocks our body runs on when we shift our eating habits. Mahan says it's like "putting them on a different time zone than the master circadian clock in the brain [which controls sleep]."

A good night's rest can not only keep you fresh for the day, but also help you remain on track for your weight loss goals. Some quick tips for improving your sleep -

- Be careful with your caffeine intake (how much and when)
- Stay hydrated
- Avoid alcohol before bed
- Avoid spicy or fatty foods before bed
- Cut back on sugar

As always, if you are having severe trouble sleeping, speak with your doctor and get to the root of the problem.

Follow Body Positivity Movements & Organizations

Our social media feeds have surged with posts advocating for body positivity in the past few years. There are people out there who assume that the movement is about promoting obesity and unhealthy lifestyles. But in reality, it is about accepting yourself and your body the way it is. The Body Positivity movement works to assure people that there is nothing wrong with them no matter how much certain sectors of society tell them otherwise. In the larger scheme of things, this movement is about more than just loving yourself. It provides you a space to question ideas about our bodies that are in reality sexist, racist, fatphobic, ableist, etc. As the movement gained more and more traction over the years, people across the globe were liberated from the sick body ideals society had stuffed down their throats.

Health at Every Size is another great initiative that encourages people to prioritize their health for the sake of their wellbeing and not to live up to the white, Western beauty standards that are always imposed on us. The organization also recognizes the fact that how we manage our health and take care of our body depends on many factors such as our environment, our economic standards, and social standing amongst other things.

Find Your Worth Outside Your Body

Almost every second person today has a hard time accepting their body image. And while body image issues are not technically a mental health issue, it can trigger one. How you see yourself impacts your mental health quite a lot and that often leads to negative self-talk. Many studies attest to the fact that those with a higher body dissatisfaction are more likely to have a poor quality of life, mental distress, develop eating disorders, etc. On the other hand, those who are satisfied with their body are living a more healthy, happy life. A majority of the time your body issues stem from lack of self-esteem, confidence, social media, abuse, bullying, mental health concerns, family relations, friendship, and a multitude of other factors. But no matter how much you diet and exercise, your physical appearance can only satisfy you so much. Those chiseled abs, shredded love handles, and snatched waists will soon be a thing of the past as you age. And if your self-worth depends on just your physical appearance, honey, you're in for a lifetime of disappointment.

Sometimes, what you see in the mirror is a reflection of how you feel on the inside. Living in a society that nurtures Western beauty ideals, it can be almost impossible to ignore the negative voice in our heads. You should be able to feel good in your body without having to drastically change it for society. Here are some active steps you can take to help yourself develop a more positive outlook on your health, your body, and yourself:

- Establish your go to people to talk to about body issues
- If need be, speak to a health professional
- Clean out your social media of any platforms/organizations that speak the diet culture language
- Follow positive influencers
    - Instagram: @theshirarose, @stephanieyeboah, @louisegreen_bigfitgirl, @scarrednotscared, @mynameisjessamyn, @kai_wes, @ragenchastain
- Be mindful of the type of media you consume
- Complain to the Advertising Standards Authority about any ads that preach a certain body type of diet culture mentality
- Model healthy eating habits, positive self-talk, encourage discussion of body image, nurture an active life, etc. at home
- Be careful with the language you use to discuss bodies

AFTERWORD

We all have to remember that life is not about getting the perfect body. Every size and shape is beautiful, and worthy of love and success. Instead of driving yourself crazy standing on the scale, focus on making healthy choices every day. If you do that, you will find your own radiance and confidence. The rules on this list are a guide to help you find success on your own journey towards the best you possible. And remember this is not a punishment but a lifestyle choice, so choose what works for you.